I0420329

Essential Oils for Weight Loss

Lose Weight and Feel Great with this Essential Oils Guide!

Proven Tips and Tricks to Lose Weight NOW with Essential Oils!

Recipes Included!

Table of Contents:

Introduction

I want to thank you and congratulate you for downloading the book, *"Essential Oils for Weight Loss: Lose Weight and Feel Great with this Essential Oils Guide! Proven Tips and Tricks to Lose Weight NOW with Essential Oils! Recipes Included! "*

This book contains proven steps and strategies on how to effectively lose weight in a stress-free manner following the instructions, and using tips and recipes outlined in this book.

Obesity has become a huge concern which is why weight loss has received a lot of attention in recent times, not only among health buffs, but also among fitness enthusiasts, the medical community, and even the beauty industry. It has, in fact, become a multi-billion dollar industry. Diet fad after diet fad have continuously gained worldwide followers despite the seemingly never-ending new concepts and approaches riding on peoples' insatiable quest for what will work in a less demanding way.

Now come essential oils; and as usual, there are naysayers and people who swear by it. Essential oils have suddenly claimed a prominent and unique position in the field of weight management, though, primarily because they also targets the one area that is often overlooked – the psychological or emotional aspect. A lot of people usually fail to complete their training and diet regimens because of a lack of motivation and the whole weight loss ordeal just being more stressful, and essential oils aims to make it easier.

What is noteworthy with these products is that they go back a long long way; they were already used in ancient cultures.. In the same vein, there were recent scientific studies that prove the effectiveness of essential oils in weight management. These things helped trigger its growing popularity worldwide. If you are looking for a more effective and natural yet relaxing weight loss program that is affordable and will not wreak havoc on your schedule, essential oils give you a reason to be truly optimistic and hopeful.

Thanks again for downloading this book. I hope you enjoy it!

☐ Copyright 2015 by Spirit Publishing- All rights reserved.

This document is geared towards providing exact and reliable information in regards to the topic and issue covered. The publication is sold with the idea that the publisher is not required to render accounting, officially permitted, or otherwise, qualified services. If advice is necessary, legal or professional, a practiced individual in the profession should be ordered.

- From a Declaration of Principles which was accepted and approved equally by a Committee of the American Bar Association and a Committee of Publishers and Associations.

In no way is it legal to reproduce, duplicate, or transmit any part of this document in either electronic means or in printed format. Recording of this publication is strictly prohibited and any storage of this document is not allowed unless with written permission from the publisher. All rights reserved.

The information provided herein is stated to be truthful and consistent, in that any liability, in terms of inattention or otherwise, by any usage or abuse of any policies, processes, or directions contained within is the solitary and utter responsibility of the recipient reader. Under no circumstances will any legal responsibility or blame be held against the publisher for any reparation, damages, or monetary loss due to the information herein, either directly or indirectly.

Respective authors own all copyrights not held by the publisher.

The information herein is offered for informational purposes solely, and is universal as so. The presentation of the information is without contract or any type of guarantee assurance.

The trademarks that are used are without any consent, and the publication of the trademark is without permission or backing by the trademark owner. All trademarks and brands within this book are for clarifying purposes only and are the owned by the owners themselves, not affiliated with this document.

Chapter 1: What are Essential Oils?

Essential oils are highly concentrated aromatic compounds in hydrophobic liquid form. They are extracted from plant leaves, roots, flowers, fruits, and seeds. A single drop can have immense impact on health. Distillation through steaming is the usual way essential oil is produced by separating the oil from the plant's water-based compounds.

Because it is extremely concentrated, producing it is akin to pooling all the plant's powerful healing properties in one substance as one expert opined. It has been a prominent feature particularly in Indian, Egyptian, Chinese, Roman, and Greek cultures in terms of spiritual, medicinal, and cosmetic uses since ancient times. It has been in constant use undergoing changes, innovation, and improvement for almost 6,000 years already.

One well-known example is India's 5,000-year old Ayurveda system of holistic healing. It has recently gone through a kind of renaissance that made it a much sought-after form of alternative remedy among natural healing enthusiasts. The ancient Egyptians, of course, are particularly famous for the use of essences, aromatic resins, and balms for cosmetic and medicinal application, and particularly for embalming as exemplified by the legendary Egyptian mummy.

The use of essential oils in modern times, particularly the upsurge in the popularity of aromatherapy got its most important boost in an accidental laboratory explosion experienced by French chemist, René-Maurice Gattefossé, in 1928. In his desperation to alleviate the burn that his hands suffered, he soaked it in the nearest container with a friendly-looking substance. The substance turned out to be lavender oil which fortuitously healed his hands quickly without scarring.

He decided to study lavender oil and its possible uses for treating skin problems like burns, wounds, and infections for the original purpose of helping injured soldiers during World War I. That launched the chemist into a lifelong study and experimentation for aromatic or essential oils which started a worldwide trend. He actually coined the term aromatherapy. This gave birth to the science of aromatherapy. Through massage therapists and beauticians, the use of essential oils spread all over Europe. Eventually, it crossed the Atlantic and began to be popular in the United States in the 1980s where the oils found its way into different lotions, candles, and fragrances.

Today, there are many trained professionals that make use of the essential oils in their vocation such as aromatherapists, nutritionists, massage therapists, physical therapists, and even doctors of natural medicine. The past few decades, more advanced and sustained scientific researches on the manifold benefits of essential oils have shown very promising results. These include mood altering and curative effects, as well as physiological benefits.

One of the most important recent discoveries or

rediscoveries about essential oils that has the world of physical fitness and natural health remedies all agog is weight loss. The multi-level marketing (MLM) community is, in fact, one of the quickest to jump into the fray. Online health purveyors have flooded the internet with their own findings and recommendations. So if you are one of the millions worldwide who had gone through all those diet fads in the past 2 decades, you can learn from the advent of essential oils too.

Being all natural, it has no known significantly harmful side effects. One unique aspect brought about by essential oils in weight loss research is the added emphasis on brain conditioning in shedding extra pounds. Getting healthy and getting fit have become a key measure for over-all quality of life to many. In the following sections, how these oils work, which essential oils are most effective, and corresponding recipes will be discussed.

Just a word of caution, though. Essential oils can be very handy in matters that promote weight loss.

These include curbing appetite, improving digestion, balancing mood, boosting metabolism, and controlling blood sugar levels. But it is not a miracle weight management remedy. It needs to be combined with balanced diet and regular exercise for maximum results.

Chapter 2: How Essential Oils Work

Using the human brain to accomplish weight loss includes both psychological and physiological aspects that take their cue from the brain's supreme controlling function over your body. In the case of aromatic compounds like essential oils, it is about how smell impacts the brain and thus various body functioning.

Consider how we feel when we smell things that remind us of camping with loved ones, family reunions, and provincial summer vacations. Like the scent of smoke from crackling dried leaves or the roaring bonfire in evening gatherings. Such smells can kindle nostalgia and bring back pleasant memories. In effect, the brain can interpret smells as memories. It can produce soothing feelings that can influence other parts of the body to react in a certain way, like neutralizing stresses in your daily life. The brain can also be similarly impacted to promote weight loss. For instance the hypothalamus part of the brain can also be soothed to lessen distressing emotions linked to weight problems, namely, depression, fear and anger, and anxiety. Essential oils can perform the functions of antidepressants without the addictive effects.

A study by Dr. Hirsh connecting peppermint smell and weight reduction took six months and involved 3,000 people with dramatic results. Everyone involved in the study experienced a reduction in weight at 30 pounds on average with some opting out earlier because of concern for excessive weight loss. Additional similar studies conducted at the Universities of Vienna and Berlin revealed another way essential oils are causing weight loss. Some oils, it was revealed, substantially increase brain oxygen thereby dramatically impacting stress and hormone imbalance among other things. These two things alone support healthy weight loss. More findings from other studies are trickling in showing more ways essential oils are helping weight reduction.

Nowhere is this impact of essential oils more compelling than with aromatherapy. Reportedly, your nose can recognize one trillion distinct odors which instantly stimulate parts of the brain. The olfactory glands of the nose and the brain's amygdala and hippocampus can quickly interact. Depending on what scent invaded the nose, its impact on one's mental, physical, and emotional states could be very positive. Brain receptors that deal with things like pleasure, motivation, and stress levels get cues from the nose about smells that it detected.

Essential oils could help a lot in a weight loss program because a lot of the obstacles arise from psychophysiological factors. Things like depressed moods, slow metabolism, dieting fatigue, emotional eating, or lack of consistent motivation can benefit from the use of essential oils. Reducing stress helps reduce cortisol levels in your body. Stress-induced high cortisol levels are known culprit for heightened weight gain in the abdomen even in slim women. This was confirmed in a 2000 study published in the Psychosomatic Medicine journal. But a 2014 study featured in Complementary Therapies in Medicine displayed substantial decrease in salivary cortisol levels after just one aromatherapy massage.

Another study that proves certain scents could result to weight loss was done at Japan's Niigata University School of Medicine. As published in the Journal of Experimental Biology and Medicine, the study showed that the body's ability to burn fat while suppressing further weight gain can be triggered by grapefruit and lemon smell. In Korea's Wonkwang Health Science College, a 6-week research convincingly demonstrated significant reduction in the belly fat of post-menopausal women through abdominal massage using certain essential oils. In fact, an earlier study done in 2000 on aromatherapy massage helped reduce not only fat and waist size but also appetite in middle-aged women. Additionally, the study found that a blend of grapefruit, lemon, and cypress oils were far more effective in reducing belly fat compared to grapefruit oil alone. This is an important finding that must be considered in weight loss essential oil preparation.

So if you are unhappy with your belly, you can try mixing a blend recommended by one convinced promoter consisting of grapefruit, sweet orange, cypress, and juniper berry with sunflower seed oil as carrier oil for massage. A parallel explanation states that citrus oils like grapefruit, lemon, orange, and grapefruit essential oils are very effective in cleansing our metabolic pathways. This toxin-cleansing process helps in weight reduction. Also, a corollary result was that those who had more waist reduction, the citrus-cypress blend users, experienced more body image improvement. Finally, because it is more difficult for such changes to happen among post-menopausal women, it could only mean it is more likely to occur among men and women in general.

Still, most people would need some lifestyle changes, such as unhealthy eating habits, to get the best results. This is despite the proven efficacy of essential oils in shedding and maintaining weight. It is definitely good news, of course, that these oils can assist the body in burning those unsightly stored fats and eliminating toxins. But more than that, those oils can also help lessen body fluid retention, reduce food craving, fight emotional stress, and boost system metabolism which are all quite useful for weight loss.

Chapter 3: Ways to Use Essentials Oils for Weight Loss

In general, there are 5 ways in using essential oils for weight loss, namely:

1. Open the essential oil bottle and inhale the scent for at least 5 minutes by holding the container to your nose.

2. Spread the scent throughout your room using an aromatherapy diffuser

3. If you are always on the go, wear an aromatherapy necklace so you can do it anywhere.

4. Through a warm bath, put five drops of the essential oil onto it and for 30 minutes immerse in the tub.

5. Using a carrier, dilute the essential oil and massage your body or at least the part where there is a concentration of fat that needs removal.

From someone fond of concocting blends and mixes

at home comes an encouragement for you to try experimenting with your own combinations of scents based on your preferences and to have fun with it. The important thing is to attain a high healing quality for each type of oil.

There are many listings that you can actually see online when it comes to proven recipes that help you achieve general wellness. You just need to do a little checking and personal assessment to determine which ones are best for you. Below are examples that can serve as a pattern or starting points for you in formulating your own weight loss mixture:

· **Metabolism Booster Bath** - Add two tablespoons of jojoba oil, 10 drops of rosemary, 10 drops of cypress, and eight drops of grapefruit oil in a warm bath preparation.

· **Fat Breaking Rub** - Using a carrier oil, mix two drops each of cypress, peppermint, and ginger oils with 10 drops of grapefruit and five drops of rosemary. Rub it to the body gently.

- **Cellulite Reducing Massage** - Combine five drops each of grapefruit, lemon, and cypress oil with a quarter cup of almond oil. Then massage the target area in the body.

- **Craving Curtailing Lotion** - Blend 40 drops of bergamot, 24 drops of patchouli oil, a half cup of olive oil, and 80 drops of fennel. Use the solution to massage abdomen area.

- **Craving Curbing Dab** -- Use essential oils like peppermint, grapefruit, ginger, cinnamon or lemon. Suppress hunger or increase energy by dabbing a drop on your wrists.

- **Appetite Controlling Dispersion** - Mix 12 drops of ginger with 40 drops of mandarin, 12 drops of peppermint, and 20 drops of lemon. Put a few drops of the blend to your diffuser.

- **Revitalizing Soak** - Prepare a warm bath and put in it five drops each of orange, grapefruit, lemon, ginger, and sandalwood.

For abdominal massage, you can use certain techniques to achieve good results. In a circular way forming large circles, massage the oil in the abdominal area starting above the belly button moving slowly to the abdomen's left side. Do it every day or at least 5 times a week for ideal results. One precaution: Grapefruit and lemon can cause minor photo sensitivity. So do not use it right after sunlight exposure and wait three hours at least. If there are allergic reactions, stop using it.

Massage therapy has many benefits. In the area of weight loss, it increases circulation, reduces stress, and heightens lymphatic flow. In the abdomen, massage minimizes constipation and improves digestion. So a daily massage would go a long way in maximizing its benefits. A better circulation and lymphatic flow transport much needed nutrients and oxygen to all bodily cells while cleansing the body of metabolic waste, toxins, and bacteria. An additional benefit would be a body that is more efficient at controlling water retention and regulating hormones. These are important for weight loss, not to mention being better looking and healthier.

To further clarify its usage, the following are the three basic classifications of essential oil application based on certain psychophysiological principles:

1. **Topical**

Essential oils are ideal for direct skin application because it can be readily absorbed by the skin due to its small molecular size. It is an established scientific fact that for the skin to absorb a particular substance, it should have a molecular weight below 1,000m (m=weight of molecule). The chemical weight of essential oils is less than 1000m. This property enables essential oil molecules to easily enter the skin and into the blood stream where it is carried all over the body by blood. That is how it is able to impact your body internally with its therapeutic benefits.

2. <u>Aromatic</u>

Apart from the skin, the nose and lungs have also been proven adept in welcoming essential oils to the body. Apparently, these oils can also be absorbed into the bloodstream when inhaled. What facilitate this route to the body for the essential oils are the numerous blood vessels lurking in your lungs that let in the oils and then transport it around the body. The great thing with inhalation is you can simply spread the oil around your room or office using a diffuser. You can do your weight loss therapy while working at your office table, or while simply resting in your favorite chair watching TV, browsing the internet or reading your favorite book. You don't have to undress and get wet or massage any part of your body for 10 minutes or more. For specific oil and its intended benefits, you can diffuse peppermint for increased energy and focus. You can also use lavender to decrease stress, orange to lift mood, melaleuca for cleaner air, and frankincense for better meditation.

3. <u>Ingestion</u>

This is the most direct way for essential oils to enter your body and do its job, whether for weight loss or other benefits. But always remember that essentials oils are highly concentrated that it cannot be utilized even via skin in undiluted form. Otherwise, it could be harmful rather than beneficial to the user. With such concentration, it could be a powerful form of medicine in the sense that a few drops can go a long way. But it can also easily cause an overdose even though it is natural. What can give you pause when it comes to ingestion is that a topical application via skin alone is very delicate already when it comes to amount. So although most essential oils are safe for ingestion, limit yourself to 1-3 drops per glass of drinking water.

Chapter 4: Most Effective Essential Oils for Weight Loss

Following is a list of the more potent essentials oils, and the mechanisms that make them truly effective for weight loss.

Grapefruit Essential Oil

With a sweet and uplifting aroma, grapefruit oil is generally utilized as an antiseptic and disinfectant.

Main functions

- Curtails cravings of food

- Boosts metabolism which lessens fat storage

- Enhances body energy and endurance

- Minimizes abdominal fat build up

Scientific Principle

What makes grapefruit oil effective for weight loss is the active ingredient nootkatone. It acts on AMPK, an enzyme that has to do with the metabolic rate and energy levels of the body. Studies show that the interactions between AMPK and nootkatone results in the reduction in body fat and weight gain, among other things. Another research had lab rats subjected to grapefruit oil three times a week and the result was loss of weight and appetite reduction. The findings were attributed to the lipolysis action of grapefruit's primary ingredient, limolene, which breaks down and dissolves protein and body fat. It also enhances metabolism and smooth flow in the lymphatic glands which both promote weight loss.

The essential oil of the fruit comes from its peel. Being excellent lymphatic stimulant and diuretic, grapefruit essential oil is a component in a lot of cellulite cream and mixes. In effect, grapefruit is the most popular essential oil when it comes to weight loss and fat burning owing to its ability to activate the right enzymes. The nice thing about an essential oil is that its efficacy is enhanced or broadened when mixed with other essential oils. In the case of grapefruit oil, a combination with patchouli oil also reduces cravings and hunger. When you think about it, it connotes a stress-free, faster, and natural way of losing weight. When you feel a craving, either rub some in your chest or wrist or diffuse in your room or office.

Other actions attributed to grapefruit oil that help manage weight are its prevention of bloating and water retention. It also helps in getting the fatty acids to circulate in your blood stream which helps in breaking down fat converting it to energy for your body use. One new research revealed that its reduction of cholesterol level and lipid peroxidation in your body is one way limolene is promoting weight loss. Even its ability to help cleanse the body of toxins which contribute to weight gain is getting recognized. Grapefruit oil has vitamin C that contains lycopene which in turn assists in cleansing the lymphatic system, necessary for toxin removal. Toxins that are not flushed out are stored as body fat.

How to Use

You can massage with it specific parts of your body after mixing it with a carrier such as virgin coconut oil or virgin olive oil. If cold, make sure to warm the oil a little bit by soaking its bottle in a container with hot water. Otherwise it can cause shock and stress. The massage should be done in a circular clockwise movement for about 30 minutes. Do not wash it right away after the massage leaving it for a few hours for maximum effect so you need to plan you activities around it if you need to take a bath. Try doing it for at least six weeks, twice a day, as done in the 2007 Korean study.

Another way to benefit from it is to add a drop or two in a refreshing glass of water and drinking it prior to breakfast. This morning ritual will help you to flush out more toxins and lose excess fat. It's very good for fat burning and toxin cleansing. Make sure to buy quality or food grade essential oil for internal consumption. Finally, you can prepare a blend that you should take before breakfast. You can include in this five drops each of orange juice, ginger oil, lemon oil, and sandalwood.

And the by the way, if you are into other body enhancing activities, you can incorporate this fat busting massage in your daily health routine. It definitely is better if such a routine includes eating healthy food and exercise. Grapefruit oil is also able to block weight gain by minimizing the production of cortisol. Cortisol is a stress-induced substance that triggers your body to produce insulin that causes fat storage. Less cortisol, less insulin, less fat stored. Likewise, one factor that causes problems in weight management is insulin resistance. And one thing that promotes insulin resistance is a carbohydrate and sugar-rich diet that is exacerbated by the addition of omega-6 vegetable oils based on the Standard American Diet. Grapefruit is effective in achieving hormonal balance which is important in weight reduction.

When to Use

You can be a little adventurous in your use of grapefruit oil for massaging away unwanted fat or cellulite. For those undergoing hormone fluctuations, be it peri-menopause or menopause, you might adjust your usage based on your observation of differences in how weight or even bulges are distributed in your body. And even with body functions unchanging, chemical compounds like xenoestrogen can accumulate in your body causing weight gain by tampering with your metabolism. All these essential oil applications, by the way, apply to both men and women. Do the massage in the morning with the grapefruit oil mixed with a carrier oil. A study at Munich's Technische Universitaet and the University of Vienna points to the superior quality of olive oil as carrier as its scent also helps lower calorie consumption among people.

Apart from both massage and drinking which should be done in the morning, another time you can use the grapefruit essential oil is during bath time. Just add 5 drops into a warm bath plus a cup of apple cider vinegar for greater impact. Disperse oil with your hands and soak for about 30 minutes.

Lemon Essential Oil

Lemon oil scent has a distinct characteristic that evokes a clean feeling though with some tangy nuance. It is processed from the peel through cold press method.

Main functions:

- Suppresses weight gain

- Increases energy

- Enhances mood

Scientific principle:

Like grapefruit, lemon oil is also powered by limonene which is good for fat burning. In the same study findings extolling the virtues of grapefruit oil for weight loss, its tandem with lemon was found to be more effective in increasing lipolysis. Lemon has many benefits to the body but one of its most relevant functions is the capacity to raise the body's norepinephrine levels, a stress hormone and neurotransmitter. This hormone boosts heart rate and blood flow that helps muscle to work better and speedier. If you are on a muscle-straining workout routine, lemon can act as pain reliever.

Again like grapefruit, lemon oil assists the body in flushing out toxins that cause weight gain by stimulating the liver. It also has weight loss-promoting polyphenols. By the way, did you know that intestinal parasites have a major role in weight gain? Well, lemon oil can eliminate such parasites. Likewise, it also enhances energy, metabolism, and digestion which are helpful in fat breakdown. In combination with peppermint, lemon oil is effective in suppressing appetite.

How to Use

Regular massage with lemon oil, especially around the cellulite areas will help one get rid of toxins that are stored in the body as fat. By regularly cleansing the body of toxins, one becomes healthier. In the morning, mix one to two drops of lemon oil with the water you drink because it is also a good detoxifier. Make sure you are using oil of high and food grade quality. Or just inhale by holding the opened bottle in your nose or diffusing it in your room or office. A simpler inhaler would be a cotton ball with a few drops of lemon essential oil. Before a meal or snack, gently inhale the vapors to curtail appetite and overeating. You can put in a small zip bag if traveling. Daily massage, on the other hand, is good for eliminating accumulated cellulite and the stored toxins in fat cells.

Lemon oil, like grapefruit contains not only limonene but vitamins and minerals that promote weight loss through improve digestive health, body detox, better metabolism, and appetite suppression.

These functions seem to be served repeatedly with these oils' different features but it only enhances its usefulness.

Peppermint Essential Oil

Peppermint oil which has menthol exudes a minty scent, of course, but with the freshness and intensity that is calming and cooling.

Main functions:

- Enhances energy and mental alertness

- Elevates mood that prevents weight inducing stress

- Aids digestion and better metabolism

- Reduces appetite which in weight loss is self-explanatory

Scientific principle

Peppermint is one of those essential oils with ancient roots as a continuous go-to remedy for indigestion. Its weight loss function gets a lot of push from its 70% menthol component enabling it to be a good muscle relaxant, reduce bloating, and improve rate of food passage in the body by enhancing the flow of bile. Its mood calming effect minimizes weight-inducing stress.

Peppermint oil's characteristic as a natural appetite suppressant is very useful in weight management. In 2008, a study was conducted on peppermint's impact on appetite entitled Effects of Peppermint Scent on Appetite Control and Caloric Intake. The results show that inhaling peppermint oil every two hours lowers hunger levels and significantly reduces calorie consumption. A part of your brain makes you feel full and peppermint oil greatly encourages that feeling whenever you eat. This was validated in a recent scientific research on the effectiveness of peppermint oil that found people who inhaled the oil having much less craving for food than those who did not.

Also, it was proven to be effective for giving relief to people suffering from stomach upset. Additionally, peppermint like lemon and grapefruit contains nutrients and vitamins such as Vitamin C that contribute to over-all body wellbeing.

How to Use

You can use peppermint either by drinking, by inhaling, or by soaking in a bath. In drinking, add one to two drops of high quality food grade oil to one glass of drinking water. It works in no small measure in stunting appetite. You can also breathe in the scent by holding the bottle to your nose and or inhaling from small cotton ball with the oil before eating. You would feel less desirous of eating. Finally, 5 to 10 drops of peppermint oil to your warm bath water can give you a rejuvenating soak which is best done in the morning.

There is another type of eating disorder, however, the overeater. Some people don't know when to stop once they have started eating. They don't think of whether they are full already or not yet. They allow themselves to be guided by the continuing urge to eat, whatever the reason. Peppermint oil is effective in countering the urge to overeat. It gives a full feeling after a meal while providing energy. Finally, it also improves digestive health which again is key to weight loss. The Chicago Smell and Taste Treatment and Research Institute found that peppermint and lemon essential oils are tops in helping curb appetite and weight loss.

Cinnamon Essential Oil

An inviting and sweet fragrance is what sets cinnamon apart from other essential oils. It is extracted from the leaves or inner bark of the Cinnamomum tree.

Main functions:

- Improves insulin sensitivity that enhances metabolism and fat breakdown.

- Regulates blood sugar levels that helps weight loss

- Reduces inflammation thereby lessening stress

Main principle

Cinnamon prevents insulin resistance in the body that leads to excessive weight gain. This condition happens when body cells stop reacting to insulin resulting in a confusion on function that goads your body to erroneously store fat instead of burning it. The harmful result is not only weight gain but also inability to lose weight. However, this does not only involve the weight issue; it can also lead to Type 2 diabetes. Cinnamon helps increase brain insulin insensitivity and blood glucose uptake rate. About 25% of Americans are actually affected by this condition that includes abdominal obesity and insulin resistance so it is not something minor. Relatedly, the body fat of genetically obese people contains inflammatory cells whose production cinnamon oil has inhibited and is important for thwarting weight gain.

Cinnamon is actually considered the second most effective essential oil for weight management. Because of its blood glucose regulation function, cinnamon helps balance blood sugar which overtime helps in weight loss and curbing sugar cravings. Imbalances in sugar level can trigger weight gain and overeating. But adding cinnamon oil to food and drink hinders release of glucose into the blood. In the same vein, it also helps cleanse the body of toxin-harboring fat. Cinnamon oil possesses other outstanding attributes. It gives you a sense of being full, for one. Its advantage is that it prevents weight gain which is superior to and easier than losing weight, of course. Cinnamon also aids in preventing accumulation of fatty acid by helping convert sugar into energy instead of storing it as fat. Finally, it promotes better blood circulation, increased metabolism, and inflammation prevention which are all conducive to weight loss.

How to Use

For inhaling, breathe in cinnamon essential oil before eating to restrain your appetite. Try using a cotton ball with a few drops of the oil. For drinking, try mixing honey with a glass of water and add one or two drops of cinnamon oil into it. Drink it upon waking up in the morning or before going to bed at night to avoid nighttime cravings. Overeating is especially bad at night because the body in bed is no longer active to burn it. Again, ensure your supply of high quality or food grade cinnamon essential oil for internal use.

Bergamot Essential Oil

The bergamot essential oil makes a good blend with orange characterized by a tangy and sweet scent with hints of spiciness.

Main functions:

- Boosts mood or anti-depressant

- Increases energy

Scientific principle

The usefulness of bergamot in weight management also comes by way of psychology. A lot of people resort to overeating, though maybe unconsciously, in moments of anxiety and depression. It may give you a temporary high but eventually it becomes a vicious cycle of binge eating and emotional lows adding more unwanted pounds. Bergamot oil has been proven to be a good remedy for that problem.

In a study on the effectiveness of bergamot oil aromatherapy, it was reported that in just 15 minutes bergamot had caused improvement in emotional condition and level of energy plus instant physiological benefits. Those who inhaled bergamot had substantially lower signs of stress as evidenced by much lower cortisol level than those who did not. In fact, bergamot is an Italian citrus fruit that is traditionally eaten to relieve stress. Conversely, the bergamot essential oil is best for people whose weight problem stemmed from stress-induced overeating. Combining with lavender essential oil gives bergamot more efficacy in this function.

Additionally, bergamot is quite useful in burning sugar, oxidizing fat, boosting metabolism, and keeping out bad cholesterol. What makes this possible is bergamot's high level of polyphenols, similar to green tea. One other unique feature of bergamot is its ability to hinder an enzyme that promotes higher blood sugar levels and as trigger for speedier breakdown of sugar and fat.

How to Use

Add one or two drops of bergamot essential oil on a cloth and inhale to relieve stressful moments and neutralize the desire to eat to quell your emotions. You will feel better and energized. For a more revitalizing drink, put in one to two drops to a mixture of coconut milk and honey. As for body massage, use olive oil or coconut oil as carrier focusing on the feet and neck area. You can also make use of a good relaxing warm bath by adding several drops of bergamot oil into it in the morning and you're off to a good start. It will help you through the day.

Fennel Essential Oil

Fennel essential oil is extracted from fennel seeds and emits a sweet and earthy aroma.

Main Functions:

- Improves digestion

- Suppresses appetite

- Hinders weight gain

- Improves sleep quality

Scientific principle:

The use of fennel for suppressing appetite goes back to the middle ages especially during fasting. Intrigued by this bit of history, modern scientists performed an experiment on rats involving fennel oil aromatherapy. One major finding shows fewer calories consumed and faster food digestion among rats that inhaled fennel oil twice a day for a period of eight weeks. The sleep improvement function of fennel, however, comes from its melatonin content. But although it is famous for its role in promoting restful sleep, melatonin also helps control weight gain by favoring more the production of beige fat or fat that burns as energy rather than white fat or fat stored for energy.

Ginger Essential Oil

What makes ginger oil tick as a weight loss substance is its active ingredient gingerols. Gingerols is proven to be effective in minimizing disease-causing intestinal inflammation and, hence, improving absorption of vitamins and minerals. This action enhances cellular energy in the body and facilitates weight reduction. These three factors of better nutrient absorption, improved digestion, and reducing inflammation are essential in losing weight. In addition, ginger oil curtails craving for sweets or sugar.

These characteristics were confirmed in a 2003 scientific study on the essential oil published in the Indian Journal of Physiology and Pharmacology. In this research, ginger oil exhibited significant anti-inflammatory, anti-nociceptive, and antioxidant characteristics. Inflammation is, of course, now accepted as playing a key part in obesity. Finally, the gingerols in ginger serves to boost thermogenesis which enhances metabolism in the body. You can employ the usage methodology mentioned in other essential oils here for ginger oil.

Orange Essential Oil

Orange oil's effectiveness as a weight management agent originates from its large amount of Vitamin C. This ingredient has strong antioxidant and anti-inflammatory properties. The weight loss or weight gain prevention function comes in the form of detoxifying and cleansing the lymphatic system because of such properties. As mentioned previously, toxins that cannot go out of the body because of clogged lymph canals add more pounds because it is stored in excess fats. So in general, orange essential oil is beneficial because of its role as fat burner, metabolism stimulant, and lymphatic system detoxifier. You can use the methods employed in other essential oils in the use of this oil.

Oregano Essential Oil

Oregano essential oil is also anti-inflammatory due to its active ingredient, carvacrol. Inflammation's role in obesity takes place in the white adipose tissue of the body. Just like other essential oils, oregano helps in preventing weight gain by alleviating inflammation. Equally important, oregano oil neutralizes your food cravings by increasing your body's dopamine levels. For usages involving ingestion, massage, inhalation, and soaking, you can refer to other essential oils here.

Chapter 5: Additional Essential Oils Weight Loss Recipes

<u>Abdominal Fat-Burning Massage Oil</u>:

· Prepare two ounces of virgin olive oil, as carrier for the essential oils, in a cup.

· Put in 5 drops each of lemon, cypress, and grapefruit essential oils to the cup.

· Transfer the blend in a glass bottle, closed it, and gently shake to mix the contents uniformly.

· Two times every day, massage your abdominal area with a small amount of the oil blend for maximum result.

<u>Essential Oil Rejuvenating Massage Blend (1 oz.)</u>

<u>Ingredients and Supplies</u>:

- grapefruit essential oil, 4 drops

- cypress essential oil, 4 drops

- juniper berry essential oil, 4 drops

- sweet orange essential oil, 4 drops

- sage essential oil, 1-2 drops

- virgin olive oil or virgin coconut oil, 1 oz.

- dark colored massage bottle, 1 piece

Note: if sweet orange is not available, you can use ginger, lemon or fennel.

Directions:

Place the carrier oil (virgin olive or coconut) into the dark massage bottle. Add to it the essential oil drops in the list. Shake gently for uniform blending before each use. Store out of direct heat and sunlight to maintain quality.

Precaution:

When using aromatherapy on children or the elderly

use a much lower amount (0.5 to 1 ½% concentration only) based on the age of the person. Also, do not use sage oil on a child.

Assumption:

There are 600 drops of essential oil per ounce in a bottle with a euro-dropper. The size of drops can vary, so when in doubt, measure using milliliters instead of drops to be accurate. Use 1 ml. (.9 ml to be exact) of essential oil for every 30 ml. of massage oil to get a 3% concentration.

Cellulite Buster Bath Blend

Prepare a warm bath and add in a mixture of 5 drops each of ginger, orange, lemon, grapefruit, and sandalwood essential oils plus 1 cup raw apple cider vinegar. To avoid evaporation, refrain from adding essential oils with running water. Immerse yourself in the bath for around half an hour.

Fat-Burning Capsule Mix

To curb your appetite and burn fat faster, take one capsule with a glass of water daily after breakfast. Always use food grade essential oils for internal consumption.

Ingredients (per capsule):

- peppermint essential oil, 2 drops

- grapefruit essential oil, 2 drops

- lemon essential oil, 2 drops

- coconut oil (virgin) as carrier, 12 drops

Instruction:

Mix the ingredients and place in a capsule. For more mixes, put greater quantity of the ingredients in a vial using the exact proportion of the essential oils and the carrier. Then package in more capsules based on the average content per capsule of six drops of the essential oils plus 12 drops of the carrier. To keep it fresh, keep the capsules in the fridge.

Chapter 6: Safety Precautions

Because essential oils are extremely concentrated, make sure it does not come into contact with your skin, eyes or mucous membranes in its pure form, meaning without the carrier. It would be good to use gloves while mixing. Lavender is an exception because it is good for the skin. Wash with soap and water if it gets in your skin. Dip your eyes in a basin of water immediately if it gets in there for several minutes. Get medical help if those measures fail.

Likewise, be aware of contraindication for specific essential oils. For children, the elderly, and the pregnant women, do not use sage oil. During pregnancy juniper berry oil is also not suitable. In contrast, grapefruit, cypress, and orange stand as the safest. Consult an expert when you are not sure.

As mentioned, always use a carrier to dilute the essential oils before topical application or direct use in the skin. Test it before full application to prevent allergic reaction. One way is to do a small skin patch test on the intended area. If there is no adverse reaction after 24 hours you can do the full application on all targeted body parts. Otherwise, discontinue using it on your body. Finally, there are essential oils especially those from citrus fruits which do not react well with light or phototoxic. Do not get exposed to direct sunlight for 12-18 hours after using such types of oil. Lastly, oils like peppermint, lemon and frankincense can be taken with water. But others like clove and oregano should be diluted and cannot be ingested for more than 1 week.

Conclusion

Thank you again for downloading this book!

I hope this book was able to help you to learn revolutionary new steps for fulfilling your weight management and other health goals.

The next step is to apply what you have learned here in your life.

Finally, if you enjoyed this book, then I'd like to ask you for a favor, would you be kind enough to leave a review for this book on Amazon? It'd be greatly appreciated!

Thank you and good luck!

www.ingramcontent.com/pod-product-compliance
Lightning Source LLC
Chambersburg PA
CBHW071129280526
45787CB00003B/1222